50 Acne Erasing Juice Recipes:

Quickly Reduce Visible Acne without Creams or Medicine

By

Joe Correa CSN

COPYRIGHT

This publication is designed to provide accurate and authoritative information in regard to the subject matter covered. It is sold with the understanding that neither the author nor the publisher is engaged in rendering medical advice. If medical advice or assistance is needed, consult with a doctor. This book is considered a guide and should not be used in any way detrimental to your health. Consult with a physician before starting this nutritional plan to make sure it's right for you.

ACKNOWLEDGEMENTS

This book is dedicated to my friends and family that have had mild or serious illnesses so that you may find a solution and make the necessary changes in your life.

50 Acne Erasing Juice Recipes:

Quickly Reduce Visible Acne without Creams or Medicine

By

Joe Correa CSN

CONTENTS

Copyright

Acknowledgements

About The Author

Introduction

50 Acne Erasing Juice Recipes: Quickly Reduce Visible Acne without Creams or Medicine

Additional Titles from This Author

ABOUT THE AUTHOR

After years of Research, I honestly believe in the positive effects that proper nutrition can have over the body and mind. My knowledge and experience has helped me live healthier throughout the years and which I have shared with family and friends. The more you know about eating and drinking healthier, the sooner you will want to change your life and eating habits.

Nutrition is a key part in the process of being healthy and living longer so get started today. The first step is the most important and the most significant.

INTRODUCTION

50 Acne Erasing Juice Recipes: Quickly Reduce Visible Acne without Creams or Medicine

By Joe Correa CSN

Having clear and beautiful skin is a precious gift but unfortunately most people tend to suffer from acne breakouts. Every year, people spend millions and millions of dollars searching for the perfect or easy solution to clean their skin. But in the end, most of them are left dissapointed with the same problem they had in the first place. Without any doubt, there is no miracle solution that will clean your skin overnight and help you get rid of acne. Whatever your skin condition is, you will have to follow some basic rules that have been proven to be the right formula for clean and beautiful skin.

Regular facial hygiene is the first step you'll have to take to remove impurities, extra oil from your skin, and dead skin cells that cause this problem in the first place. Cleaning your face with warm water twice a day is a proven method to reduce acne and will you keep you skin clean. However, make sure not to use harsh soaps as they will probably cause more damage than good and may even irritate your delicate skin. After you have washed your face, gently dry it with a clean towel and avoiding harsh scrubbing.

Dermatologists agree that a gentle moisturizer will neutralize the damage most acne product cause by minimizing the dryness and skin peeling. When buying these products, make sure to read the labels.

As I said earlier, these basic steps are the first thing to do for your skin but the secret lies in your diet. All doctors and nutritionists agree that a clear and glowing skin comes from within. The right amount of vitamins, minerals, and fluids will literally clean your entire body, including your skin. Foods like berries, tomatoes, mint, nuts, watercress, fennel, grapes, beetroot, avocado, and kale are among the top skin cleaning ingredients that should be on your table every day. This is why a good, nutrient-rich juice is the right way to go!

For this reason, I have created this wonderful collection of acne preventing and eliminating juice recipes. These juices are based on the foods mentioned above and will give your body exactly what it needs to clean itself and eliminate your acne problem once and for all. Try them all and start having skin that looks and feels great. You deserve it!

50 ACNE ERASING JUICE RECIPES: QUICKLY REDUCE VISIBLE ACNE WITHOUT CREAMS OR MEDICINE

1.   Pear Ginger Juice

Ingredients:

1 small pear, chopped

1 small ginger knob, peeled

1 cup of pumpkin, cubed

1 small green apple, cored

1 oz of water

Preparation:

Wash the pear and cut in half. Remove the core and cut into small chunks. Set aside.

Peel the ginger and cut into small pieces. Set aside.

Peel the pumpkin and cut lengthwise in half. Scoop out the seeds and cut into small cubes. Fill the measuring cup and reserve the rest in the refrigerator.

Wash the apple and cut in half. Remove the core and cut into bite-sized pieces. Set aside.

Now, combine pumpkin, apple, pear, and ginger in a juicer and process until juiced. Transfer to a serving glass and stir in the water.

Add some ice and serve immediately.

Nutrition information per serving: Kcal: 167, Protein: 2.4g, Carbs: 50.7g, Fats: 0.6g

2.   Apple Basil Juice

Ingredients:

1 medium-sized Granny Smith's apple, cored

1 cup of fresh basil, chopped

2 cups of broccoli, chopped

1 cup of fennel, chopped

1 oz of water

Preparation:

Wash the apple and cut lengthwise in half. Remove the core and chop into small pieces. Set aside.

Rinse the basil thoroughly under cold running water. Drain and torn into small pieces. Set aside.

Wash the broccoli and trim off the outer leaves. Chop into small pieces and fill the measuring cup. Reserve the rest for later. Set aside.

Trim off the fennel stalks and outer wilted layers. Wash and chop the fennel into bite-sized pieces. Fill the measuring cup and reserve the rest for later. Set aside.

Now, combine apple, basil, broccoli, and fennel in a juicer and process until juiced. Transfer to a serving glass and stir in the water.

Refrigerate for 5 minutes before serving.

Nutrition information per serving: Kcal: 140, Protein: 7.7g, Carbs: 41.8g, Fats: 1.3g

3.   Blueberry Lemon Juice

Ingredients:

1 cup of blueberries

1 whole lemon

2 medium red bell peppers, chopped

1 large wedge of honeydew melon

Preparation:

Wash the blueberries under cold running water. Drain and set aside.

Peel the lemon and cut lengthwise in half. Set aside.

Wash the bell peppers and cut in half. Remove the seeds and chop into small pieces. Set aside.

Cut the honeydew melon lengthwise in half. Scoop out the seeds using a spoon. Cut the large wedges and peel them. Cut into small chunks and place in a bowl. Wrap the rest of the melon in a plastic foil and refrigerate.

Now, process blueberries, lemon, bell peppers, and honeydew melon in a juicer.

Transfer to serving glasses and add some ice.

Serve immediately.

Nutritional information per serving: Kcal: 202, Protein: 5.5g, Carbs: 59.3g, Fats: 1.7g

4.   Apple Orange Juice

Ingredients:

1 medium-sized Granny Smith's apple, cored

1 medium-sized orange, peeled

1 cup of celery, chopped

1whole kiwi, peeled

1 tbsp of liquid honey

¼ tsp of ginger, ground

Preparation:

Wash the apple and cut lengthwise in half. Remove the core and cut into bite-sized pieces. Set aside.

Peel the orange and divide into wedges. Cut each wedge in half and set aside.

Wash the celery and chop into small pieces. Fill the measuring cup and reserve the rest for later. Set aside.

Peel the kiwi and cut lengthwise in half. Set aside.

Now, combine celery, kiwi, apple, and orange in a juicer and process until juiced. Transfer to a serving glass and stir in the honey and ginger.

Refrigerate for 5 minutes before serving.

Enjoy!

Nutrition information per serving: Kcal: 172, Protein: 3.5g, Carbs: 51.2g, Fats: 1.1g

5. Apple Celery Juice

Ingredients:

1 small Granny Smith's apple, cored

1 large celery stalk, chopped

1 tsp of aloe juice

1 cup of cucumber, sliced

1 medium-sized banana, sliced

Preparation:

Wash the apple and cut in half. Remove the core and cut into bite-sized pieces. Set aside.

Wash the celery stalk and chop into bite-sized pieces. Set aside.

Wash the cucumber and cut into thin slices. Fill the measuring cup and reserve the rest for later. Set aside.

Peel the banana and cut into chunks. Set aside.

Now, combine apple, cucumber, banana, and celery in a juicer. Process until juiced.

Transfer to a serving glass and stir in the aloe juice.

Add some crushed ice and refrigerate for 5 minutes before serving.

Nutrition information per serving: Kcal: 174, Protein: 2.7g, Carbs: 50.3g, Fats: 0.8g

6.   Tomato Basil Juice

Ingredients:

1 large tomato, chopped

1 cup of fresh basil, torn

1 large cucumber, sliced

½ tsp of dried oregano, ground

1 oz of water

Preparation:

Wash the tomato and place it in a medium bowl. Cut into small pieces and reserve the juice while cutting. Set aside.

Wash the basil thoroughly and torn with hands. Set aside.

Wash the cucumber and cut into thick slices. Set aside.

Now, process tomato, basil, and cucumber in a juicer. Transfer to serving glasses and stir in the reserved tomato juice and water.

Sprinkle with dried oregano for some extra taste and serve immediately.

Nutritional information per serving: Kcal: 67, Protein: 4.3g, Carbs: 18.6g, Fats: 0.8g

7.   Sweet Apricot Pear Juice

Ingredients:

1 cup of apricots, pitted and halved

1 small pear, chopped

1 tbsp of liquid honey

1 small Delicious apple, cored

1 whole lemon, peeled and halved

1 cup of fresh mint, torn

Preparation:

Wash the apricots and cut each lengthwise in half. Remove the pits and fill the measuring cup. Reserve the rest in the refrigerator for some other juice.

Wash the pear and cut in half. Remove the core and cut into small pieces. Set aside.

Wash the apple and cut lengthwise in half. Remove the core and chop into bite-sized pieces. Set aside.

Peel the lemon and cut lengthwise in half. Set aside.

Rinse the mint thoroughly under cold running water. Drain and torn into small pieces. Set aside.

Now, combine apricots, pear, apple, lemon, and mint in a juicer and process until well juiced. Transfer to a serving glass and add some ice before serving.

Enjoy!

Nutrition information per serving: Kcal: 217, Protein: 4.9g, Carbs: 68.5g, Fats: 1.5g

8.   Apple Coconut Juice

Ingredients:

1 large Granny smith apple, peeled and cored

½ cup of pure coconut water, unsweetened

1 cup of pumpkin cubes

1 large banana, peeled

¼ tsp of nutmeg, ground

1 tbsp of coconut sugar

Preparation:

Wash the apple and remove the core. Cut into bite-sized pieces and set aside.

Peel the pumpkin and cut in half. Scoop out the seeds using a spoon. Cut one large wedge and peel it. Cut into small chunks and set aside. Reserve the rest for later.

Peel the banana and cut into chunks. Set aside.

Now, process pumpkin, banana, and apple in a juicer. Transfer to serving glasses and stir in the coconut water, coconut sugar, and nutmeg.

Refrigerate for 30 minutes before serving.

Nutritional information per serving: Kcal: 338, Protein: 4.6g, Carbs: 97.8g, Fats: 1.4g

9.   Grapefruit Cauliflower Juice

Ingredients:

1 whole grapefruit, peeled

1 cup of cauliflower, chopped

1 large orange, peeled

1 cup of pineapple chunks

¼ cup of pure coconut water, unsweetened

Preparation:

Peel the grapefruit and orange and divide into wedges. Set aside.

Trim off the outer leaves of cauliflower. Wash it and cut into small pieces. Reserve the rest in the refrigerator.

Cut the top of a pineapple and peel it using a sharp knife. Cut into small chunks. Reserve the rest of the pineapple in a refrigerator.

Now, process pineapple, grapefruit, orange, and cauliflower in a juicer.

Transfer to serving glasses and stir in the pure coconut water.

Add few ice cubes and serve immediately.

Nutritional information per serving: Kcal: 247, Protein: 6.5g, Carbs: 74g, Fats: 1g

10.   Guava Cucumber Juice

Ingredients:

1 large guava, peeled

1 large cucumber

1 ripe avocado, pitted and peeled

1 large lime, peeled

2 oz of coconut water

Preparation:

Peel the guava and cut into small chunks. Set aside.

Wash the cucumber and cut into thick slices. Set aside.

Peel the avocado and cut in half. Remove the pit and cut into chunks. Set aside.

Peel the lime and cut lengthwise in half. Set aside.

Now, process avocado, guava, cucumber, and lime in a juicer. Transfer to serving glasses and stir in the coconut water.

Add some ice cubes or refrigerate for 5 minutes.

Nutrition information per serving: Kcal: 352, Protein: 7.6g, Carbs: 41.6g, Fats: 30.3g

11.   Celery Cherry Juice

Ingredients:

1 cup of celery, chopped

1 cup of cherries, pitted

1 cup of watermelon, diced

1 small ginger knob, peeled

1 oz of water

¼ tsp of cinnamon, ground

Preparation:

Wash the celery and cut into small pieces. Fill the measuring cup and reserve the rest for later. Set aside.

Rinse the cherries under cold running water using a colander. Drain and cut each in half. Remove the pits and set aside.

Cut the watermelon in half. Cut one large wedge and wrap the rest in a plastic foil and refrigerate. Dice the wedge and remove the pits. Fill the measuring cup and set aside.

Peel the ginger knob and cut into small pieces. Set aside.

Now, combine watermelon, celery, cherries, and ginger knob in a juicer and process until juiced. Transfer to a serving glass and stir in the water and cinnamon. Add some ice and serve immediately.

Nutrition information per serving: Kcal: 143, Protein: 3.4g, Carbs: 40.2g, Fats: 0.7g

12.   Apple Strawberry Juice

Ingredients:

1 small apple, cored

2 large strawberries, chopped

2 large bananas, peeled and chunked

1 cup of fresh mint, chopped

2 oz of water

Preparation:

Wash the apple and cut in half. Remove the core and cut into bite-sized pieces. Set aside.

Wash the strawberries and remove the stem. Cut into bite-sized pieces and set aside.

Peel the bananas and cut into small chunks. Set aside.

Wash the mint and roughly chop it. Fill the measuring cup and set aside.

Now, combine apple, strawberries, bananas, and mint in a juicer and process until juiced. Transfer to a serving glass and stir in the water.

Add some ice and serve immediately.

Nutrition information per serving: Kcal: 294, Protein: 4.5g, Carbs: 86.1g, Fats: 1.4g

13. Grapefruit Parsley Juice

Ingredients:

1 whole grapefruit, peeled

4 cups of parsley, chopped

1 cup of cantaloupe, diced

2 cups of mustard greens, torn

¼ cup of water

Preparation:

Peel the grapefruit and divide into wedges. Set aside.

Wash the mustard greens and parsley. Torn with hands and set aside.

Cut the cantaloupe in half. Scoop out the seeds and flesh. Cut two wedges and peel them. Chop into chunks and set aside. Reserve the rest of the cantaloupe in a refrigerator.

Now, process cantaloupe, mustard greens, grapefruit, and parsley in a juicer.

Transfer to serving glasses and stir in the water.

Add some ice and serve immediately.

Nutritional information per serving: Kcal: 206, Protein: 13.5g, Carbs: 59.3g, Fats: 3g

14.   Cranberry Blueberry Juice

Ingredients:

1 cup of fresh cranberries

1 cup of fresh blueberries

3 medium Zestar apples, cored

1 cup of fresh kale, torn

1 tbsp of liquid honey

Preparation:

Combine cranberries and blueberries in a colander and wash under cold running water. Drain and set aside.

Wash the apples and remove the core. Cut into bite-sized pieces and set aside.

Wash the kale thoroughly and torn with hands. Set aside.

Now, process cranberries, blueberries, apple, and kale in a juicer.

Transfer to serving glasses and stir in the honey. Add some ice or refrigerate before serving.

Nutrition information per serving: Kcal: 368, Protein: 5.6g, Carbs: 106g, Fats: 2.2g

15.   Radish-Swiss Chard Juice

Ingredients:

1 large radish, chopped

1 cup of chard, torn

1 cup of asparagus

1 cup of avocado, chopped

1 large honeydew melon wedge

¼ cup of pure coconut water, unsweetened

Preparation:

Wash the radish and trim off the green parts. Cut into small pieces and set aside.

Wash the chard thoroughly and torn with hands. Set aside.

Wash the asparagus and trim off the woody ends. Set aside.

Peel the avocado and cut in half. Remove the pit and cut into chunks. Set aside.

Cut the honeydew melon lengthwise in half. Scoop out the seeds using a spoon. Cut the large wedges and peel them. Cut into small chunks and place in a bowl. Wrap the rest of the melon in a plastic foil and refrigerate.

Now, process radish, chard, asparagus, avocado, and melon in a juicer.

Transfer to serving glasses and refrigerate 10 minutes before serving.

Nutritional information per serving: Kcal: 275, Protein: 8g, Carbs: 35.2g, Fats: 21,9g

16.   Mango Lemon Juice

Ingredients:

1 cup of mango, cubed

1 large lemon, peeled

1 cup of fresh cherries, pitted

1 cup of watermelon, cubed

1 tbsp of liquid honey

2 oz of water

Preparation:

Peel the mango and cut into small chunks. Set aside.

Peel the lemon and cut lengthwise in half. Set aside.

Wash the cherries under cold running water. Drain and cut in half. Remove the pits and set aside.

Cut the watermelon lengthwise. For one cup, you will need about 1 large wedge. Peel and cut into chunks. Remove the seeds and set aside. Reserve the rest of the melon for some other juices.

Now, process cherries, mango, lemon, and watermelon in a juicer.

Transfer to serving glasses and add few ice cubes before serving.

Nutrition information per serving: Kcal: 288, Protein: 4.6g, Carbs: 68.3g, Fats: 1.3g

17.   Carrot Cucumber Juice

Ingredients:

1 large carrot, peeled and sliced

1 cup of cucumber, sliced

1 large wedge of honeydew melon, peeled and cubed

1 cup of Swiss chard, torn

1 small ginger knob, peeled

¼ tsp of turmeric, ground

2 oz of water

Preparation:

Wash and peel the carrot. Cut into thin slices and set aside.

Wash the cucumber and cut into thin slices. Fill the measuring cup and reserve the rest for later. Set aside.

Cut melon lengthwise in half. Scoop out the seeds and then wash. Cut one large wedge and peel it. Cut into small cubes and set aside.

Rinse the Swiss chard thoroughly under cold running water. Drain and torn into small pieces. Set aside.

Peel the ginger knob and cut into small pieces. Set aside.

Now, combine melon, Swiss chard, carrot, and cucumber in a juicer and process until juiced. Transfer to a serving glass and stir in the turmeric and water.

Refrigerate for 10 minutes before serving.

Nutrition information per serving: Kcal: 92, Protein: 2.6g, Carbs: 25.7g, Fats: 0.5g

18.   Pumpkin Carrot Juice

Ingredients:

1 cup of pumpkin, cubed

2 large carrots, sliced

2 cups of Brussels sprouts, halved

1 small ginger knob, peeled and chopped

1 oz of water

Preparation:

Cut the pumpkin in half and scoop out the seeds. For one cup, you'll need about one large wedge. Cut and peel. Chop into bite-sized pieces and fill the measuring cup. Wrap the rest of the pumpkin in a plastic foil and reserve in the refrigerator.

Wash and peel the carrots. Cut into thin slices and set aside.

Wash the Brussels sprouts and trim off the outer wilted layers. Cut each sprout in half and set aside.

Peel the ginger knob and chop it into small pieces. Set aside.

Now, combine pumpkin, carrots, Brussel sprouts, and ginger in a juicer and process until juiced. Transfer to a serving glass and stir in the water.

Add some ice and serve immediately.

Nutrition information per serving: Kcal: 127, Protein: 8.5g, Carbs: 38.2g, Fats: 1.1g

19. Carrot Apple Juice

Ingredients:

1 large carrot, sliced

1 small Granny Smith's apple, cored and chopped

1 cup of mango, chunked

1 oz of coconut water

Preparation:

Wash and peel the carrot. Cut into bite-sized pieces and set aside.

Wash the apple and cut in half. Remove the core and cut into bite-sized pieces. Set aside.

Peel the mango and cut into chunks. Fill the measuring cup and reserve the rest for later.

Now, combine carrot, apple, and mango in a juicer. Process until juiced. Transfer to a serving glass and stir in the coconut water. Add some crushed ice and serve immediately.

Enjoy!

Nutrition information per serving: Kcal: 179, Protein: 2.6g, Carbs: 51.2g, Fats:1.1g

20.   Banana Milk Juice

Ingredients:

1 large banana, peeled

2 tbsp of milk

2 cups of blueberries

1 cup of black grapes

1 cup of fresh mint, torn

¼ tsp of cinnamon, ground

Preparation:

Wash the banana and cut into thin slices. Set aside.

Place the blueberries in a colander. Rinse well under cold running water and drain. Set aside.

Wash the grapes and remove the stems. Fill the measuring cup and reserve the rest in the refrigerator. Set aside.

Wash the mint thoroughly under cold running water. Drain and torn into small pieces. Set aside.

Now, combine blueberries, grapes, mint, and banana in a juicer and process until juiced. Transfer to a serving glass and stir in the milk and cinnamon.

Refrigerate for 5 minutes before serving.

Nutrition information per serving: Kcal: 326, Protein: 6.2g, Carbs: 93.4g, Fats: 2.1g

21. Kale Strawberry Juice

Ingredients:

1 cup of fresh kale, torn

1 cup of strawberries, fresh

½ tsp of ginger, ground

1 lemon, peeled

Preparation:

Wash the kale thoroughly and torn with hands. Set aside.

Wash the strawberries under cold running water. Drain and set aside.

Peel the lemon and cut lengthwise in half. Set aside.

Combine kale, strawberries, and lemon in a juicer and process until juiced.

Transfer to a serving glass and add some ice cubes before serving.

Enjoy!

Nutritional information per serving: Kcal: 120, Protein: 5.9g, Carbs: 38.6g, Fats: 1.8g

22.   Tomato Mustard Green Juice

Ingredients:

1 medium-sized Roma tomato, chopped

1 cup of mustard greens, torn

2 cups of Romaine lettuce, chopped

1 cup of parsley, torn

1 whole cucumber, sliced

¼ tsp of turmeric, ground

¼ tsp of salt

Preparation:

Wash the tomato and place in a bowl. Chop into bite-sized pieces and reserve the tomato juice while cutting. Set aside.

Combine mustard greens and parsley in a large colander. Rinse well and drain. Torn into small pieces and set aside.

Rinse the lettuce thoroughly under cold running water. Chop into small pieces and set aside.

Wash the cucumber and cut into thin slices. Set aside.

Now, combine lettuce, tomato, mustard greens, parsley, and cucumber in a juicer and process until juiced. Transfer to a serving glass and stir in the turmeric, salt, and reserved tomato juice.

Refrigerate for 10 minutes before serving.

Enjoy!

Nutrition information per serving: Kcal: 85, Protein: 7.6g, Carbs: 25.3g, Fats: 1.6g

23.　Beet Apple Juice

Ingredients:

1 cup of beets, sliced

1 small Granny Smith's apple, cored

1 cup of fresh kale, torn

1 cup of cantaloupe, cubed

¼ tsp of ginger, ground

Preparation:

Wash the beets and trim off the green ends. Cut into thin slices and fill the measuring cup. Reserve the rest for some other juice.

Wash the apple and cut lengthwise in half. Remove the core and cut into bite-sized pieces. Set aside.

Rinse the kale thoroughly under cold running water. Drain and torn into small pieces. Set aside.

Cut the cantaloupe in half. Scrape out the seeds and cut one large wedge. Peel and chop into small pieces. Fill the measuring cup and wrap the rest in a plastic foil. Refrigerate for later.

Now, combine beets, apple, kale, and cantaloupe in a juicer and process until juiced. Transfer to a serving glass and stir in the ginger.

Add some ice and serve immediately.

Nutrition information per serving: Kcal: 181, Protein: 7g, Carbs: 51.1g, Fats: 1.4g

24.   Orange Apple Juice

Ingredients:

1 large orange, peeled

1 small Granny Smith's apple, cored

1 cup of papaya, chopped

1 cup of fresh mint, torn

1 tbsp of fresh basil, torn

Preparation:

Peel the orange and divide into wedges. Cut each wedge in half and set aside.

Wash the apple and cut in half. Remove the core and cut into bite-sized pieces. Set aside.

Wash and peel the papaya. Cut lengthwise in half and scoop out the seeds. Cut into bite-sized pieces and fill the measuring cup. Reserve the rest in the refrigerator.

Rinse the mint and basil thoroughly under cold running water. Drain and torn into small pieces. Set aside.

Now, combine orange, apple, papaya, mint, and basil in a juicer and process until juiced. Transfer to a serving glass and add some ice.

Serve immediately and enjoy!

Nutrition information per serving: Kcal: 199, Protein: 4.1g, Carbs: 60.1g, Fats: 1.1g

25. Pumpkin Cinnamon Juice

Ingredients:

10 ozof sweet pumpkin chunks

½ tsp of cinnamon, freshly ground

1 cup of avocado chunks

¼ cup of water

Preparation:

Peel the pumpkin and cut in half. Scoop out the seeds using a spoon. Cut one large wedge and peel it. Cut into small chunks and set aside. Reserve the rest for later.

Peel the avocado in half. Remove the pit and cut into small chunks. Set aside.

Now, combine avocado and pumpkin in a juicer and process until juiced.

Transfer to serving glasses and stir in the water and cinnamon.

Add some ice before serving and enjoy!

Nutritional information per serving: Kcal: 256, Protein: 5.3g, Carbs: 27.8g, Fats: 22.3g

26. Leek Asparagus Juice

Ingredients:

1 whole leek, chopped

2 medium-sized asparagus spears

1 cup of avocado, cubed

1 medium-sized zucchini

3 tbsp of water

Preparation:

Wash the leek and cut into small pieces. Set aside.

Wash the asparagus and trim off the woody ends. Cut into small pieces and set aside.

Peel the avocado and cut lengthwise in half. Remove the core and cut into small cubes. Fill the measuring cup and reserve the rest in the refrigerator.

Peel the zucchini and cut into bite-sized pieces. Set aside.

Now, combine avocado, zucchini, leek, and asparagus in a juicer and process until juiced. Transfer to a serving glass and stir in the water.

Refrigerate for 10 minutes before serving.

Enjoy!

Nutrition information per serving: Kcal: 277, Protein: 22.9g, Carbs: 32.7g, Fats: 22.9g

27.   Blackberry Cinnamon Juice

Ingredients:

1 cup of blackberries

¼ tsp of cinnamon, ground

1 cup of cantaloupe, chopped

1 large orange, peeled

1 cup of fresh mint, torn

Preparation:

Place the blackberries in a colander and rinse well. Drain and set aside.

Cut the cantaloupe in half. Scrape out the seeds and cut one large wedge. Peel and chop into small pieces. Fill the measuring cup and wrap the rest in a plastic foil. Refrigerate for later.

Peel the orange and divide into wedges. Cut each wedge in half and set aside.

Rinse the mint under cold running water and drain. Torn into small pieces and set aside.

Now, combine and blackberries, cantaloupe, orange, and mint in a juicer and process until juiced. Transfer to a serving glass and stir in the cinnamon.

Add some ice and refrigerate for 5 minutes before serving.

Nutrition information per serving: Kcal: 157, Protein: 5.9g, Carbs: 51.9g, Fats: 1.5g

28.   Apricot Cucumber Juice

Ingredients:

1 cup of apricots, pitted

1 large cucumber

1 large peach, pitted

1 large apple, cored

1-inch piece of ginger root

Preparation:

Wash the peach and apricots. Cut in half andremove the pit. Cut into bite-sized pieces and set aside.

Wash the cucumber and cut into thick slices. Set aside.

Wash the apple and remove the core. Cut into bite-sized pieces and set aside.

Peel the ginger and set aside.

Now, combine apricots, peach, cucumber, apple, and ginger in a juicer. Process until juiced. Transfer to serving glasses and add some ice.

Serve immediately.

Nutrition information per serving: Kcal: 257, Protein: 6.7g, Carbs: 73.3g, Fats: 1.8g

29. Carrot Cabbage Juice

Ingredients:

1 cup of carrots, sliced

1 cup of purple cabbage, chopped

1 cup of cauliflower, chopped

1 cup of collard greens, chopped

Preparation:

Wash the cauliflower and trim off the outer leaves. Cut into bite-sized pieces and fill the measuring cup. Reserve the rest for later.

Wash and peel the carrots. Cut into thin slices and fill the measuring cup. Set aside.

Combine cabbage and collard greens in a colander. Wash thoroughly under cold running water and slightly drain. Chop into small pieces and set aside.

Now, combine carrots, cabbage, cauliflower, and collard greens in a juicer and process until juiced. Transfer to a serving glass and refrigerate for 5 minutes before serving.

Nutrition information per serving: Kcal: 138, Protein: 5.3g, Carbs: 40.3g, Fats: 0.8g

30.   Celery Cucumber Juice

Ingredients:

2 celery stalks

1 large cucumber

3 large tomatoes

2 large carrots, sliced

1 bunch of fresh spinach

1 large bell pepper

Preparation:

Wash the celery and cucumber and chop into small pieces. Set aside.

Wash the tomatoes and place them in a bowl. Cut into small pieces and reserve the tomato juice while cutting. Set aside.

Wash the carrots and slice into a bowl with tomatoes.

Wash the bell pepper and cut in half. Remove the seeds and chop into small pieces.

Wash the spinach thoroughly and roughly chop it. Set aside.

Now, process tomatoes, carrots, celery, cucumber, spinach, and bell pepper in a juicer. Transfer to serving glasses and add the juices from the bowl.

Garnish with some fresh mint, but this is optional.

Refrigerate for 5 minutes before serving.

Enjoy!

Nutritional information per serving: Kcal: 248, Protein: 3.71g, Carbs: 70.5g, Fats: 3.71g

31. Apple Mint Juice

Ingredients:

1 small apple, peeled and seeds removed

1 tsp of fresh mint leaves, finely chopped

1 cup of pineapple chunks

¼ tsp of nutmeg, ground

Preparation:

Wash the apple and remove the core. Cut into bite-sized pieces and set aside.

Garnish with mint leaves and refrigerate before serving.

Cut the top of a pineapple and peel it using a sharp knife. Cut into small chunks. Reserve the rest of the pineapple in a refrigerator.

Process pineapple and apple in a juicer. Transfer to a serving glasses and stir in the nutmeg. Add more water to increase the juice amount.

Nutritional information per serving: Kcal: 141, Protein: 1.5g, Carbs: 41.2g, Fats: 0.4g

32.   Orange Lettuce Juice

Ingredients:

1 large orange, peeled

1 cup of Romaine lettuce, shredded

1 cup of watermelon, peeled and seeded

1 cup of pomegranate seeds

Preparation:

Peel the orange and divide into wedges. Set aside.

Wash the lettuce thoroughly. Roughly chop it using hands and add set aside.

Cut the watermelon lengthwise. For one cup, you will need about one large wedge. Peel and cut into chunks. Remove the seeds and set aside.

Cut the top of the pomegranate fruit using a sharp knife. Slice down to each of the white membranes inside of the fruit. Pop the seeds into a medium bowl.

Now, process watermelon, orange, lettuce and pomegranate seeds in a juicer. Transfer to serving glasses and refrigerate for 5 minutes.

Nutritional information per serving: Kcal: 142, Protein: 5.2g, Carbs: 44.8g, Fats: 1.5g

33.   Parsnip Orange Juice

Ingredients:

1 cup of parsnip, sliced

1 small orange, peeled

1 large peach, peeled

3 cups of red leaf lettuce, torn

1 tsp of agave syrup

Preparation:

Wash the parsnips and cut into thick slices. Set aside.

Peel the orange and divide into wedges. Set aside.

Wash the peach and cut in half. Remove the pit and cut into bite-sized pieces. Set aside.

Wash the lettuce thoroughly and torn it using hands. Set aside.

Now, process parsnips, orange, peach, and lettuce in a juicer. Transfer to serving glasses and stir in the agave syrup.

Add some ice and serve immediately.

Nutritional information per serving: Kcal: 177, Protein: 5.2g, Carbs: 53.7g, Fats: 1.1g

34.   Carrot Parsnip Juice

Ingredients:

3 large carrots, sliced

1 cup of parsnips, sliced

2 large green apples, peeled and cored

1 basil leaf, crushed

¼ cup of water

Preparation:

Wash the carrots and parsnips and cut into thick slices. Set aside.

Wash the apples and remove the core. Cut into bite-sized pieces and set aside.

Now, combine apples, carrots, and parsnips in a juicer and process until juiced.

Transfer to serving glasses and stir in the water. Garnish with basil leaves and refrigerate before serving.

Enjoy!

Nutritional information per serving: Kcal: 332, Protein: 5.4g, Carbs: 100g, Fats: 1.6g

35.   Mango Ginger Juice

Ingredients:

1 cup of mango, chunked

1 small ginger slice

1 cup of pomegranate seeds

1 medium-sized apple, cored

¼ tsp of cinnamon, ground

1 oz of water

Preparation:

Peel the mango and cut into chunks. Fill the measuring cup and reserve the rest in the refrigerator. Set aside.

Peel the ginger slice and chop into small pieces. Set aside.

Cut the top of the pomegranate fruit using a sharp paring knife. Slice down to each of the white membranes inside of the fruit. Pop the seeds into a measuring cup and set aside.

Wash the apple and cut lengthwise in half. Remove the core and cut into small pieces. Set aside.

Now, combine pomegranate seeds, apple, mango, and ginger in a juicer and process until juiced. Transfer to a serving glass and stir in the cinnamon and water.

Refrigerate for 5 minutes before serving.

Nutrition information per serving: Kcal: 227, Protein: 3.6g, Carbs: 64.1g, Fats: 1.9g

36.   Cucumber Spinach Juice

Ingredients:

1 large cucumber, sliced

1 cup of fresh spinach, torn

1 cup of pineapple chunks

1 cup of apricots

1 whole lemon

½ cup of raw broccoli, chopped

½ cup of pure coconut water

Preparation:

Wash the cucumber and chop into thick slices. Set aside.

Peel the lemon and cut lengthwise in half. Set aside.

Combine spinach and broccoli in a colander and wash under cold running water. Drain and roughly chop. Set aside.

Cut the top of a pineapple and peel it using a sharp knife. Cut into small chunks. Reserve the rest of the pineapple in a refrigerator.

Wash the apricots and cut in half. Remove the pit and chop into chunks. Set aside.

Now, process cucumber, lemon, spinach, pineapple, apricots, and broccoli in a juicer. Transfer to serving glasses and stir in the coconut water.

Add some ice and serve immediately.

Nutritional information per serving: Kcal: 218, Protein: 10g, Carbs: 64g, Fats: 1.9g

37. Lime Swiss Chard Juice

Ingredients:

1 whole lime, peeled

1 cup of chard, torn

1 cup of mango chunks

1 cup of beet greens, torn

½ cup of coconut water, unsweetened

Preparation:

Peel the lime and cut lengthwise in half. Set aside.

Combine chard and beet greens in a colander and wash under cold running water. Drain and torn with hands. Set aside.

Peel the mango and cut into small chunks. Set aside.

Now, combine lime, chard, mango, and beet greens in a juicer. Transfer to serving glasses and stir in the coconut water.

Add some ice or refrigerate for 5 minutes.

Enjoy!

Nutritional information per serving: Kcal: 108, Protein: 3.8g, Carbs: 33g, Fats: 0.8g

38.　Pepper Broccoli Juice

Ingredients:

1 small red bell pepper, seeded

1 small green bell pepper, seeded

1 small yellow bell pepper, seeded

1 cup of broccoli

1 cup of fresh kale

1 oz of water

Preparation:

Wash the bell peppers and cut in half. Remove the seeds and chop into small pieces. Set aside.

Wash the broccoli and kale in a colander under cold running water. Chop into small pieces and set aside.

Now, process peppers, broccoli, and kale in a juicer. Transfer to serving glasses and add a pinch of Cayenne pepper if you like it spicier. However, this is optional.

Serve immediately.

Nutritional information per serving: Kcal: 114, Protein: 8.7g, Carbs: 31.5g, Fats: 1.7g

39.   Apple Artichoke Juice

Ingredients:

1 Granny Smith apple, peeled and cored

1 large artichoke, chopped

1 cup of mustard greens, chopped

1 cup of Brussels sprouts

½ tsp of cinnamon, freshly ground

½ cup of pure coconut water, unsweetened

1 tsp of agave nectar

Preparation:

Wash the apple and remove the core. Cut into bite-sized pieces and set aside.

Using a sharp knife, trim off the outer leave of the artichoke. Cut into small pieces and set aside.

Wash the mustard greens and chop with hands. Set aside.

Wash the Brussels sprouts and trim off the outer layers. Set aside.

Now, process mustard greens, apple, artichoke, and Brussels sprouts in a juicer.

Transfer to serving glasses and stir in the cinnamon, coconut water, and agave nectar.

Add some ice and serve immediately.

Nutritional information per serving: Kcal: 195, Protein: 13.7g, Carbs: 63.4g, Fats: 1.3g

40.   Cucumber Turmeric Juice

Ingredients:

1 cup of cucumber, sliced

¼ tsp of turmeric, ground

1 cup of crookneck squash, cubed

1 cup of pumpkin, chopped

¼ tsp of salt

2 tbsp of water

Preparation:

Wash the cucumber and cut into thin slices. Fill the measuring cup and reserve the rest in the refrigerator.

Cut the squash lengthwise in half. Using a teaspoon, scoop out the seeds and clean it inside. Peel and cut into small cubes. Fill the measuring cup and wrap the rest in a plastic foil and refrigerate.

Peel the pumpkin and cut lengthwise in half. Scoop out the seeds and cut into small cubes. Fill the measuring cup and reserve the rest in the refrigerator.

Now, combine cucumber, squash, and pumpkin in a juicer and process until juiced. Transfer to a serving glass and stir in the turmeric, salt, and water.

Refrigerate for 5 minutes before serving.

Nutrition information per serving: Kcal: 73, Protein: 4.1g, Carbs: 19.3g, Fats: 0.9g

41.   Almond Honey Juice

Ingredients:

1 large banana, peeled

3 large red oranges, peeled

½ cup of almond milk, sugar-free

1 tbsp of honey, raw

1 tbsp of fresh mint leaves, finely chopped

Preparation:

Peel the banana and cut into small chunks. Set aside.

Peel the oranges and divide into wedges. Set aside.

Process banana and oranges in a juicer. Transfer to serving glasses and stir in the almond milk and honey.

Garnish with mint and refrigerate for 5 minutes before serving.

Enjoy!

Nutritional information per serving: Kcal: 411, Protein: 11g, Carbs: 95g, Fats: 3.1g

42.   Guava Swiss Chard Juice

Ingredients:

1 cup of pineapple chunks

1 whole guava, chopped

2 cups of chard, chopped

2 whole lemons, peeled

½ cup of coconut water, unsweetened

Preparation:

Wash the guava and cut into chunks. If you are using large fruit, reserve the rest for some other recipe in a refrigerator.

Wash the chard thoroughly under cold running water and set aside.

Cut the top of a pineapple and peel it using a sharp knife. Cut into small chunks. Reserve the rest of the pineapple in a refrigerator.

Peel the lemons and cut lengthwise in half. Set aside.

Now, process guava, chard, pineapple, and lemons in a juicer. Transfer to serving glasses and stir in the coconut water.

Add some ice and serve immediately.

Nutritional information per serving: Kcal: 130, Protein: 4.8g, Carbs: 43g, Fats: 1.2g

43. Mustard Green Apple Juice

Ingredients:

1 cup of mustard greens, chopped

1 small Granny Smith's apple, cored

1 large wedge of honeydew melon, chopped

1 cup of fresh mint, chopped

1 oz of water

Preparation:

Combine mint and mustard greens in a colander and wash thoroughly. Slightly drain and chop into small pieces. Set aside.

Cut the melon in half. Cut one large wedge and peel the peel it. Cut into small pieces and set aside. Wrap the rest of the melon in a plastic foil and refrigerate for later.

Wash the apple and cut lengthwise in half. Remove the core and cut into bite-sized pieces. Set aside.

Now, combine mint, mustard greens, melon, and apple in a juicer and process until juiced.

Transfer to a serving glass and stir in the water. Refrigerate for 5 minutes before serving.

Nutrition information per serving: Kcal: 139, Protein: 4.1g, Carbs: 40.5g, Fats: 0.9g

44.   Carrot Cabbage Juice

Ingredients:

1 cup of carrots, chopped

2 cups of green cabbage, shredded

2 kiwis, peeled

1 whole grapefruit, peeled

1 tbsp of honey, raw

Preparation:

Wash the carrots and cut into small pieces. Set aside.

Wash the cabbage thoroughly and roughly chop it using hands. Set aside.

Peel the kiwis and cut in half. Set aside.

Wash the grapefruit and cut into chunks. Set aside.

Now, process carrots, cabbage, kiwis, and grapefruit in a juicer. Transfer to serving glasses and stir in the honey.

Add some ice cubes and serve immediately.

Nutritional information per serving: Kcal: 219, Protein: 6.9g, Carbs: 69g, Fats: 1.5g

45.   Carrot Cucumber Juice

Ingredients:

1 large carrot, sliced

1 cup of cucumber, sliced

1 cup of sweet potatoes, chunked

1 ginger knob, sliced

2 oz of water

Preparation:

Wash and peel the carrot. Cut into thin slices and set aside.

Wash the cucumber and cut into thin slices. Fill the measuring cup and reserve the rest for later.

Peel the potato and cut into small chunks. Fill the measuring cup and reserve the rest for later. Set aside.

Peel the ginger knob and cut into thin slices. Set aside.

Now, combine potato, ginger, carrot, and cucumber in a juicer and process until juiced transfer to a serving glass and stir in the water.

Nutrition information per serving: Kcal: 132, Protein: 3.2g, Carbs: 36.6g, Fats: 0.4g

46.　Cucumber Cantaloupe Juice

Ingredients:

1 large cucumber

1 cup of cantaloupe, cubed

1large honeydew melon wedge

1 cup of watermelon, seeded

1 tbsp of liquid honey

1 tbsp coconut water

Preparation:

Wash the cucumber and cut into thick slices. Set aside.

Cut the cantaloupe in half. Scoop out the seeds and flesh. Cut two wedges and peel them. Chop into chunks and set aside. Reserve the rest of the cantaloupe in a refrigerator.

Cut the honeydew melon lengthwise in half. Scoop out the seeds using a spoon. Cut one large wedge and peel. Cut into small chunks and place in a bowl. Wrap the rest of the melon in a plastic foil and refrigerate.

Cut the watermelon lengthwise. For one cup, you will need about 1 large wedge. Peel and cut into chunks.

Remove the seeds and set aside. Reserve the rest of for some other juices.

Now, process cucumber, cantaloupe, honeydew melon, and watermelon in a juicer.

Transfer to serving glasses and stir in the honey and coconut water. Add some ice before serving.

Enjoy!

Nutritional information per serving: Kcal: 201, Protein: 3.4g, Carbs: 57.6g, Fats: 0.8g

47.   Pineapple Mint Juice

Ingredients:

1 cup of pineapple, chunked

1 cup of fresh mint, torn

1 cup of cucumber, sliced

1 whole guava, chopped

1 oz of water

Preparation:

Cut the top of the pineapple and peel it using a sharp paring knife. Peel it and cut into small pieces. Set aside.

Wash the mint and slightly drain. Torn with hands and set aside.

Wash the cucumber and cut into thin slices. Fill the measuring cup and reserve the rest in the refrigerator.

Wash and peel the guava fruit. Chop into bite-sized pieces and set aside.

Now, combine pineapple, mint, cucumber, and guava in a juicer and process until juiced. Transfer to a serving glass and stir in the water.

Refrigerate for 5 minutes before serving.

Nutrition information per serving: Kcal: 115, Protein: 3.6g, Carbs: 35.2g, Fats: 1.1g

48.   Broccoli Swiss Chard Juice

Ingredients:

1 cup of fresh broccoli, chopped

1 cup of Swiss chard, chopped

1 medium-sized artichoke, chopped

1 cup of cucumber, sliced

1 oz of water

Preparation:

Wash the broccoli and cut into small pieces. Fill the measuring cup and reserve the rest for later. Set aside.

Rinse the Swiss chard under cold running water. Slightly drain and chop into small pieces. Fill the measuring cup and reserve the rest in the refrigerator.

Trim off the outer leaves of the artichoke using a sharp paring knife. Wash it and cut into bite-sized pieces. Set aside.

Wash the cucumber and cut into thin slices. Fill the measuring cup and reserve the rest in the refrigerator. Set aside.

Now, combine artichoke, broccoli, Swiss chard, and cucumber in a juicer and process until juiced. Transfer to a serving glass and stir in the water.

Refrigerate for 5 minutes before serving.

Nutrition information per serving: Kcal: 65, Protein: 7.7g, Carbs: 22.7g, Fats: 0.6g

49. Beet Cauliflower Juice

Ingredients:

1 cup of beets, trimmed

1 cup of beet greens, chopped

1 small cauliflower head

1 cup of parsnips, chopped

2 tbsp of fresh parsley

Preparation:

Wash the beets and trim off the green parts. Cut into small pieces. Chop the greens and set aside.

Trim off the outer leaves of a cauliflower. Wash it and chop into small pieces. Set aside.

Wash the parsnips and cut into thick slices. Set aside.

Now, process parsnips, beets, beet greens, and cauliflower in a juicer.

Transfer to serving glasses and refrigerate for 5 minutes. Garnish with fresh parsley before serving.

Nutritional information per serving: Kcal: 166, Protein: 9.9g, Carbs: 52.3g, Fats: 1.5g

50.   Radish Mint Juice

Ingredients:

1 medium-sized radish, chopped

1 tbsp of fresh mint, chopped

1 cup of cantaloupe, diced

1 cup of beet greens

1 cup of cauliflower, chopped

Preparation:

Wash the radish and trim off the green parts. Cut into small chunks and set aside.

Trim off the outer leaves of cauliflower. Wash it and cut into small pieces. Reserve the rest in the refrigerator.

Soak the mint leaves in water. Let it stand for about 2-3 minutes.

Cut the cantaloupe in half. Scoop out the seeds and flesh. Cut two wedges and peel them. Chop into chunks and set aside. Reserve the rest of the cantaloupe in a refrigerator.

Wash the beet greens and torn with hands. Set aside.

Now, process cantaloupe, beet greens, radish, cauliflower and mint in a juicer.

Transfer to serving glasses and add some ice before serving.

Nutritional information per serving: Kcal: 123, Protein: 8.1g, Carbs: 37.7g, Fats: 1.1g

ADDITIONAL TITLES FROM THIS AUTHOR

70 Effective Meal Recipes to Prevent and Solve Being Overweight: Burn Fat Fast by Using Proper Dieting and Smart Nutrition

By

Joe Correa CSN

48 Acne Solving Meal Recipes: The Fast and Natural Path to Fixing Your Acne Problems in Less Than 10 Days!

By

Joe Correa CSN

41 Alzheimer's Preventing Meal Recipes: Reduce or Eliminate Your Alzheimer's Condition in 30 Days or Less!

By

Joe Correa CSN

70 Effective Breast Cancer Meal Recipes: Prevent and Fight Breast Cancer with Smart Nutrition and Powerful Foods

By

Joe Correa CSN